MW00713821

Sarah Foster

LEAN AND GREEN

COOKBOOK 2021

SNACK&PARTY

LEAN&GREEN RECIPES

65 healthy easy-to-make and
delicious recipes
for your Snacks and your Parties
that will
Slim down your Figure and
Make you Healthier

With Lean and Green Foods
and Foods to Avoid

Table of Contents

Introduction

Lean and green diet is a special variant of the low-fat diet, which further makes use of lean proteins instead of fat in promoting weight loss and improving health. Lean protein sources include skinless poultry, fish (e.g. cod and haddock), lean cuts of meat, eggs and vegetable proteins such as lentils and beans. This kind of diet improves the metabolism by increasing the metabolic rate that speeds up weight loss. It also reduces the risk of obesity, because following the lean and green diet does not increase body fat as much as low-fat diets.

The emphasis is on consuming a small amount of meat and fish that are eaten twice a day, together with other protein sources such as eggs, lentils and beans. The diet includes vegetables in addition to fruits that are rich in vitamins (e.g. carrots). The green food includes different varieties of beans like green lentils, black-eyed peas and soybeans. Lean and Green diet is one of the healthy diets that should be consumed frequently, because it complements all other healthy diets.

Recent studies show that lean diets have similar results to low fat diets in reducing body weight. The lean and green diet, however, do not show a considerable improvement in the health risk factors like blood lipids, blood pressure and insulin resistance compared to low-fat diets.

A green lean and cleanse diet, or simply green lean diet, is a diet similar to the concept of a raw food vegan diet, but with less emphasis on raw foods and more emphasis on whole foods that are nonetheless prepared in a way to ensure minimum use of energy during preparation or preservation, for example through the practice of lacto fermentation and cooking at low temperatures under 70 °C (158 °F).

When lean & green food merges with air frying, it can make this diet much easier for people to follow. Air frying food cuts the cooking time in half and makes the food more nutritious.

The Lean and Green diet is a great diet to try. It can help you lose weight and eat healthy foods in the process. The diet practically makes the body burn fats much faster than carbohydrates.

Carbs will be there too, but at far lower levels than before. Foods rich in carbohydrates are the body's primary fuel or the brain's food. (Our bodies turn carbs into glucose.) Because there are hardly any carbohydrates in this diet, the body will have to find a substitute source of energy to keep itself alive.

Once the body realizes that it does not have enough carbohydrates to cover the calories it burns, it turns to fat reserves to provide the required energy. Before that time, the body was using only 15% of its fat reserves for energy—the ratio changes once you start this diet. You will burn fats at a relatively faster rate than fat reserves, and after that, it will burn fat at a relatively faster rate than fat reserves. In this way, the body will find a way to get the required amount of energy from its fat stores keeping the carbs and calories under control.

If you did not change your way of living altogether and added good fats to your diet, it could take carbohydrates. In that case, you might be waiting for at least a year before you will start losing weight with this diet. For you, it is still worth doing this diet. Even if it is yearlong, you will see a great improvement in your overall health. Therefore, when you ingest fats, instead of your body storing them as fat, they are more likely to be converted into a source of energy.

As fat reserves continue to be burned, the body will tend not to gain weight. This is excellent news because fat reserves are not very easy to get rid of completely.

If you ask a nutritionist about this diet, they will recommend it without a doubt. So, if you feel like cleansing your body and starting a diet that will keep you healthy, well-fed, and slender, this diet should be your primary choice.

Engaging into lean and green diet is a good idea to improve not only our health, but also our environment. One should eat less meat products and consume more of fresh fruits and vegetables in order to lower the risk for heart disease and cancer. The latter are mostly linked with meat consumption because of the nitrates located in processed meats. Fruits and vegetables are very low-calorie foods, but they are high in fiber content and rich in vitamins.

The vegetables and fruits that deserve to be consumed are the ones that are grown organically. It is very important to avoid processed foods since they contain a high percentage of fat. Green and lean diet is also linked with the environment preservation. By cutting down meat consumption by at least 50%, we save a lot from greenhouse gas emissions. Considering that meat production requires more energy, it causes more carbon dioxide emissions compared to vegetable production. Another advantage of green and lean diet is improved health care system and lower health problems cost.

Lean and Green Foods

There are numerous categories of Lean and Green foods that you can eat while following this diet regime.

Green Foods

This section includes all kinds of vegetables that have been categorized from lower, moderate, and high in terms of carbohydrate content. One serving of vegetables should be at ½ cup unless otherwise specified.

Lower Carbohydrate - These are vegetables that contain low amounts of carbohydrates.

- A cup of green leafy vegetables, such as collard greens (raw), lettuce (green leaf, iceberg, butterhead, and romaine), spinach (raw), mustard greens, spring mix, bok choy (raw), and watercress.

- ½ cup of vegetables including cucumbers, celery, radishes, white mushroom, sprouts (mung bean, alfalfa), arugula, turnip greens, escarole, nopales, Swiss chard (raw), jalapeno, and bok choy (cooked).

Moderate Carbohydrate - These are vegetables that contain moderate amounts of carbohydrates. Below are the types of vegetables that can be consumed in moderation:

- **½ cup of any of the following vegetables** such as asparagus, cauliflower, fennel bulb, eggplant, portabella mushrooms, kale, cooked spinach, summer squash (zucchini and scallop).

Higher Carbohydrates - Foods that are under this category contain a high amount of starch. Make sure to consume limited amounts of these vegetables.

- **½ cup of the following vegetables** like chayote squash, red cabbage, broccoli, cooked collard and mustard greens, green or wax beans, kohlrabi, kabocha squash, cooked leeks, any peppers, okra, raw scallion, summer squash such as straight neck and crookneck, tomatoes, spaghetti squash, turnips, jicama, cooked Swiss chard, and hearts of palm.

Lean Foods

Leanest Foods - These foods are considered to be the leanest as it has only up to 4 grams of total fat. Moreover, dieters should eat a 7-ounce cooked portion of these foods. Consume these foods with 1 healthy fat serving.

- **Fish:** Flounder, cod, haddock, grouper, Mahi, tilapia, tuna (yellowfin fresh or canned), and wild catfish.

- **Shellfish:** Scallops, lobster, crabs, shrimp

- **Game meat:** Elk, deer, buffalo

- **Ground turkey or other meat:** Should be 98% lean

- **Meatless alternatives:**14 egg whites, 2 cups egg substitute, 5 ounces seitan, 1 ½ cups 1% cottage cheese, and 12 ounces non-fat 0% Greek yogurt

Leaner Foods - These foods contain 5 to 9 grams of total fat. Consume these foods with 1 healthy fat serving. Make sure to consume only 6 ounces of a cooked portion of these foods daily:

- **Fish:** Halibut, trout, and swordfish

- **Chicken:** White meat such as breasts as long as the skin is removed

- **Turkey:** Ground turkey as long as it is 95% to 97% lean.

- **Meatless options:** 2 whole eggs plus 4 egg whites, 2 whole eggs plus one cup egg substitute, 1 ½ cups 2% cottage cheese, and 12 ounces low fat 2% plain Greek yogurt

Lean Foods - These are foods that contain 10g to 20g total fat. When consuming these foods, there should be no serving of healthy fat. These include the following:

- **Fish:** Tuna (Bluefin steak), salmon, herring, farmed catfish, and mackerel

- **Lean beef:** Ground, steak, and roast

- **Lamb:** All cuts

- **Pork:** Pork chops, pork tenderloin, and all parts. Make sure to remove the skin

- **Ground turkey and other meats:** 85% to 94% lean

- **Chicken:** Any dark meat

- **Meatless options:** 15 ounces extra-firm tofu, 3 whole eggs (up to two times per week), 4 ounces reduced-fat skim cheese, 8 ounces part-skim ricotta cheese, and 5 ounces tempeh

Healthy Fat Servings - Healthy fat servings are allowed under this diet. They should contain 5 grams of fat and less than grams of carbohydrates. Make sure that you add between 0 and 2 healthy fat servings daily. Below are the different healthy fat servings that you can eat:

- 1 teaspoon oil (any kind of oil)

- 1 tablespoon low carbohydrate salad dressing

- 2 tablespoons reduced-fat salad dressing

- 5 to 10 black or green olives

- 1 ½ ounce avocado

- 1/3-ounce plain nuts including peanuts, almonds, pistachios

- 1 tablespoon plain seeds such as chia, sesame, flax, and pumpkin seeds

- ½ tablespoon regular butter, mayonnaise, and margarine

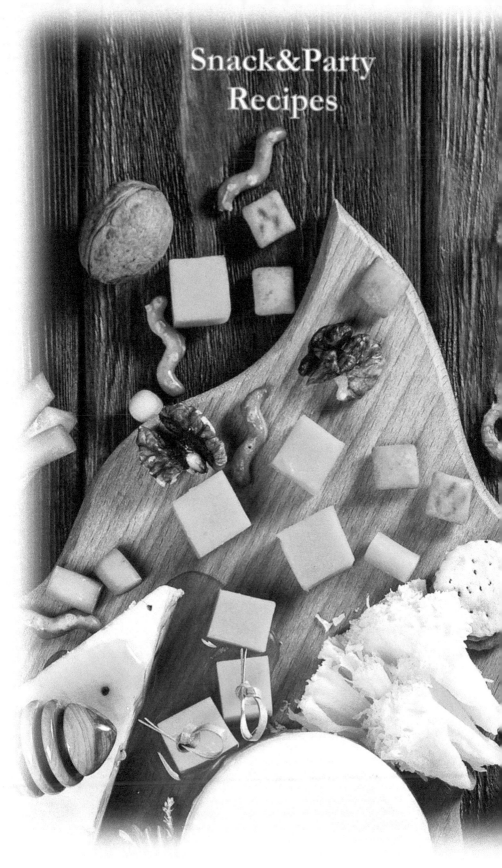

Snack&Party Recipes

1. Salmon Sandwich With Avocado and Egg

Preparation Time: 15 Minutes

Cooking Time: 10 Minutes

Servings: 4

Ingredients:

- 8 Ounces (250g) smoked salmon, thinly sliced
- 1 Medium (200g) ripe avocado, thinly sliced
- 4 Large poached eggs (about 60g each)
- 4 Slices whole wheat bread (about 30g each)
- 2 Cups (60g) arugula or baby rocket
- Salt and freshly ground black pepper

Directions:

1. Place one bread slice on a plate top with arugula, avocado, salmon, and poached egg—season with salt and pepper. Repeat the procedure for the remaining ingredients.
2. Serve and enjoy.

Nutrition:

- Calories: 310
- Fat: 18.2g
- Carbohydrates: 16.4g
- Protein: 21.3g
- Sodium: 383mg

2. Personal Pizza Biscuit

Preparation Time: 5 Minutes

Cooking Time: 15 Minutes

Servings: 1

Ingredients:

- 1 Sachet Optavia Select Buttermilk Cheddar Herb Biscuit
- 2 Tablespoons cold water
- Cooking spray
- 2 Tbsp. no-sugar-added tomato sauce
- 1/4 Cup reduced-fat shredded cheese

Directions:

1. Preheat oven to 350°F.
2. Mix biscuit and water, and spread mixture into a small, circular crust shape onto a greased, foil-lined baking sheet.
3. Bake for 10 minutes.
4. Top with tomato sauce and cheese, and cook till cheese is melted about 5 minutes.

Nutrition:

- Fats: 3.2g
- Cholesterol: 9.8mg
- Sodium: 10.5mg
- Protein: 3.6g

3. Tasty Onion and Cauliflower Dip

Preparation Time: 20 Minutes

Cooking Time: 30 Minutes

Servings: 24

Ingredients:

- 1 and ½ Cups chicken stock
- 1 Cauliflower head, florets separated
- ¼ Cup mayonnaise
- ½ Cup yellow onion, chopped
- ¾ Cup cream cheese
- ½ Teaspoon chili powder
- ½ Teaspoon cumin, ground
- ½ Teaspoon garlic powder
- Salt and black pepper to the taste

Directions:

1. Put the stock in a pot, add cauliflower and onion, heat up over medium heat, and cook for 30 minutes.
2. Add chili powder, salt, pepper, cumin, and garlic powder and stir.
3. Also, add cream cheese and stir a bit until it melts.
4. Blend using an immersion blender and mix with the mayo.

5. Transfer to a bowl and keep in the fridge for 2 hours before you serve it.

6. Enjoy!

Nutrition:

- Calories: 40 kcal
- Protein: 1.23g
- Fat: 3.31g
- Carbohydrates: 1.66g
- Sodium: 72mg

4. Marinated Eggs

Preparation Time: 2 Hours and 10 Minutes

Cooking Time: 7 Minutes

Servings: 4

Ingredients:

- 6 Eggs
- 1 and ¼ Cups of water
- ¼ Cup unsweetened rice vinegar
- 2 Tablespoons coconut aminos
- Salt and black pepper to the taste
- 2 Garlic cloves, minced
- 1 Teaspoon stevia
- 4 Ounces cream cheese
- 1 Tablespoon chives, chopped

Directions:

1. Put the eggs in a pot, add water to cover, bring to a boil over medium heat, cover and cook for 7 minutes.
2. Rinse eggs with cold water and leave them aside to cool down.
3. In a bowl, mix one cup of water with coconut aminos, vinegar, stevia, and garlic and whisk well.

4. Put the eggs in this mix, cover with a kitchen towel, and leave them aside for 2 hours, rotating from time to time.
5. Peel eggs, cut in halves, and put egg yolks in a bowl.
6. Add ¼ cup water, cream cheese, salt, pepper, and chives, and stir well.
7. Stuff egg whites with this mix and serve them.
8. Enjoy!

Nutrition:
- Calories: 289 kcal
- Protein: 15.86g
- Fat: 22.62g
- Carbohydrates: 4.52g
- Sodium: 288mg

5. Pumpkin Muffins

Preparation Time: 10 Minutes

Cooking Time: 15 Minutes

Servings: 18

Ingredients:

- ¼ Cup sunflower seed butter
- ¾ Cup pumpkin puree
- 2 Tablespoons flaxseed meal
- ¼ Cup coconut flour
- ½ Cup erythritol
- ½ Teaspoon nutmeg, ground
- 1 Teaspoon cinnamon, ground
- ½ Teaspoon baking soda
- 1 Egg
- ½ Teaspoon baking powder
- A pinch of salt

Directions:

1. In a bowl, mix butter with pumpkin puree and egg and blend well.
2. Add flaxseed meal, coconut flour, erythritol, baking soda, baking powder, nutmeg, cinnamon, and a pinch of salt and stir well.

3. Spoon this into a greased muffin pan, introduce in the oven at 350 degrees Fahrenheit and bake for 15 minutes.
4. Leave muffins to cool down and serve them as a snack.
5. Enjoy!

Nutrition:

- Calories: 65 kcal
- Protein: 2.82g
- Fat: 5.42g
- Carbohydrates: 2.27g
- Sodium: 57mg

6. Salmon Spinach and Cottage Cheese Sandwich

Preparation Time: 15 Minutes

Cooking Time: 10 Minutes

Servings: 4

Ingredients:

- 4 Ounces (125g) cottage cheese
- 1/4 Cup (15g) chives, chopped
- 1 Teaspoon (5g) capers
- ½ Teaspoon (2.5g) grated lemon rind
- 4 (2 oz. or 60g) Smoked salmon
- 2 Cups (60g) loose baby spinach
- 1 Medium (110g) red onion, sliced thinly
- 8 Slices rye bread (about 30g each)
- Kosher salt and freshly ground black pepper

Directions:

1. Preheat your griddle or Panini press.
2. Mix together cottage cheese, chives, capers, and lemon rind in a small bowl.
3. Spread and divide the cheese mixture on four bread slices. Top with spinach, onion slices, and smoked salmon.

4. Cover with remaining bread slices.
5. Grill the sandwiches until golden and grill marks form on both sides.
6. Transfer to a serving dish.
7. Serve and enjoy.

Nutrition:

- Calories: 261
- Fat: 9.9g
- Carbohydrates: 22.9g
- Protein: 19.9g
- Sodium: 1226mg

7. Sausage and Cheese Dip

Preparation Time: 10 Minutes

Cooking Time: 130 Minutes

Servings: 28

Ingredients:

- 8 Ounces cream cheese
- A pinch of salt and black pepper
- 16 Ounces sour cream
- 8 Ounces pepper jack cheese, chopped
- 15 Ounces canned tomatoes mixed with habaneros
- 1-pound Italian sausage, ground
- ¼ Cup green onions, chopped

Directions:

1. Heat up a pan over medium heat, add sausage, stir and cook until it browns.
2. Add tomatoes, mix, stir and cook for 4 minutes more.
3. Add a pinch of salt, pepper, and green onions, stir and cook for 4 minutes.
4. Spread the pepper jack cheese on the bottom of your slow cooker.
5. Add cream cheese, sausage mix, and sour cream, cover, and cook on High for 2 hours.

6. Uncover your slow cooker, stir dip, transfer to a bowl, and serve.

7. Enjoy!

Nutrition:

- Calories: 132 kcal
- Protein: 6.79g
- Fat: 9.58g
- Carbohydrates: 6.22g
- Sodium: 362mg

8. Pesto Crackers

Preparation Time: 10 Minutes

Cooking Time: 17 Minutes

Servings: 6

Ingredients:

- ½ Teaspoon baking powder
- Salt and black pepper to the taste
- 1 and ¼ Cups almond flour
- ¼ Teaspoon basil dried one garlic clove, minced
- 2 Tablespoons basil pesto
- A pinch of cayenne pepper
- 3 Tablespoons ghee

Directions:

1. In a bowl, mix salt, pepper, baking powder, and almond flour.
2. Add garlic, cayenne, and basil and stir.
3. Add pesto and whisk.
4. Also, add ghee and mix your dough with your finger.
5. Spread this dough on a lined baking sheet, introduce in the oven at 325 degrees F and bake for 17 minutes.
6. Leave aside to cool down, cut your crackers, and serve them as a snack.
7. Enjoy!

Nutrition:

- Calories: 9 kcal
- Protein: 0.41g
- Fat: 0.14g
- Carbohydrates: 1.86g
- Sodium: 2mg

9. Bacon Cheeseburger

Preparation Time: 10 Minutes

Cooking Time: 30 Minutes

Servings: 4

Ingredients:

- 1 lb. Lean ground beef
- 1/4 Cup chopped yellow onion
- 1 Clove garlic, minced
- 1 Tbsp. yellow mustard
- 1 Tbsp. Worcestershire sauce
- ½ Tsp. salt
- Cooking spray
- 4 Ultra-thin slices of cheddar cheese, cut into six equal-sized rectangular pieces
- 3 Pieces of turkey bacon, each cut into eight evenly-sized rectangular pieces
- 24 Dill pickle chips
- 4-6 Green leaf
- Lettuce leaves, torn into 24 small square-shaped pieces
- 12 Cherry tomatoes, sliced in half

Directions:

1. Pre-heat oven to 400°F.
2. Combine the garlic, salt, onion, Worcestershire sauce, and beef in a medium-sized bowl, and mix well.
3. Form the mixture into 24 small meatballs.
4. Put meatballs onto a foil-lined baking sheet and cook for 12-15 minutes.
5. Leave the oven on.
6. Top every meatball with a piece of cheese, then go back to the oven until cheese melts for about 2 to 3 minutes.
7. Let the meatballs cool.
8. To assemble bites, on a toothpick, put a cheese-covered meatball, a piece of bacon, a piece of lettuce, pickle chip, and a tomato half.

Nutrition:

- Fat: 14g
- Cholesterol: 41mg
- Carbohydrates: 30g
- Protein: 15g

10. Cheeseburger Pie

Preparation Time: 20 Minutes

Cooking Time: 90 Minutes

Servings: 4

Ingredients:

- 1 Large spaghetti squash
- 1 lb. Lean ground beef
- 1/4 Cup diced onion
- 2 Eggs
- 1/3 Cup low-fat, plain Greek yogurt
- 2 Tablespoons tomato sauce
- ½ Tsp. Worcestershire sauce
- 2/3 Cups reduced-fat, shredded cheddar cheese
- 2 oz. Dill pickle slices
- Cooking spray

Directions:

1. Preheat oven to 400°F. Slice spaghetti squash in half lengthwise; dismiss pulp and seeds.
2. Spray insides with cooking spray.
3. Place squash halves cut-side-down onto a foil-lined baking sheet, and bake for 30 minutes.

4. Once cooked, let it cool before scraping squash flesh with a fork to remove spaghetti-like strands; set aside.

5. Push squash strands in the bottom and up sides of the greased pie pan, creating an even layer.

6. Meanwhile, set up pie filling.

7. In a lightly greased, medium-sized skillet, cook beef and onion over medium heat for 8 to 10 minutes, sometimes stirring, until meat is brown.

8. Drain and remove from heat.

9. In a medium-sized bowl, whisk together eggs, tomato sauce, Greek yogurt, and Worcestershire sauce. Stir in ground beef mixture.

10. Pour pie filling over the squash crust.

11. Sprinkle meat filling with cheese, and then top with dill pickle slices.

12. Bake for 40 minutes.

Nutrition:

- Calories: 409 Cal
- Fat: 24.49g
- Carbohydrates: 15.06g
- Protein: 30.69g

11. Smoked Salmon and Cheese on Rye Bread

Preparation Time: 15 Minutes

Cooking Time: 10 Minutes

Servings: 4

Ingredients:

- 8 Ounces (250g) smoked salmon, thinly sliced
- 1/3 Cup (85g) mayonnaise
- 2 Tablespoons (30ml) lemon juice
- 1 Tablespoon (15g) Dijon mustard
- 1 Teaspoon (3g) garlic, minced
- 4 Slices cheddar cheese (about 2 oz. or 30g each)
- 8 Slices rye bread (about 2 oz. or 30g each)
- 8 (15g) Romaine lettuce leaves
- Salt and freshly ground black pepper

Directions:

1. Mix together the mayonnaise, lemon juice, mustard, and garlic in a small bowl. Flavor with salt and pepper and set aside.

2. Spread dressing on four bread slices. Top with lettuce, salmon, and cheese. Cover with remaining rye bread slices.

3. Serve and enjoy.

Nutrition:

- Calories: 365
- Fat: 16.6g
- Carbohydrates: 31.6g
- Protein: 18.8g
- Sodium: 951mg

12. Chicken and Mushrooms

Preparation Time: 10 Minutes

Cooking Time: 15 Minutes

Servings: 6

Ingredients:

- 2 Chicken breasts
- 1 Cup of sliced white champignons
- 1 Cup of sliced green chilies
- ½ Cup scallions hacked
- 1 Teaspoon of chopped garlic
- 1 Cup of low-fat cheddar shredded cheese (1-1,5 lb. grams fat / ounce)
- 1 Tablespoon of olive oil
- 1 Tablespoon of butter

Directions:

1. Fry the chicken breasts with olive oil.
2. When needed, add salt and pepper.
3. Grill the chicken breasts on a plate with a grill.
4. For every serving, weigh 4 ounces of chicken. (Make two servings, save leftovers for another meal).
5. In a buttered pan, stir in mushrooms, green peppers, scallions, and garlic until smooth and a little dark.

6. Place the chicken on a baking platter.

7. Cover with the mushroom combination.

8. Top on ham.

9. Place the cheese in a 350 oven until it melts.

Nutrition:

- Carbohydrates: 2g
- Protein: 23g
- Fat: 11g
- Cholesterol: 112mg
- Sodium: 198mg
- Potassium: 261mg

13. Chicken Enchilada Bake

Preparation Time: 20 Minutes

Cooking Time: 50 Minutes

Servings: 5

Ingredients:

- 5 oz. Shredded chicken breast (boil and shred ahead) or 99 percent fat-free white chicken can be used in a pan.
- 1 Can tomato paste
- 1 Low sodium chicken broth can be fat-free
- 1/4 Cup cheese with low-fat mozzarella
- 1 Tablespoon oil
- 1 Tbsp. of salt
- Ground cumin, chili powder, garlic powder, oregano, and onion powder (all to taste)
- 1 to 2 Zucchinis sliced longways (similar to lasagna noodles) into thin lines
- Sliced (optional) olives

Directions:

1. Add olive oil in a saucepan over medium/high heat, stir in tomato paste and seasonings, and heat in chicken broth for 2-3 min.
2. Stirring regularly to boil, turn heat to low for 15 min.

3. Set aside and cool to ambient temperature.

4. Dredge a zucchini strip through enchilada sauce and lay flat on the pan's bottom in a small baking pan.

5. Next, add the chicken a little less than 1/4 cup of enchilada sauce and mix it.

6. Attach the chicken to cover and end the baking tray.

7. Sprinkle some bacon over the chicken.

8. Add another layer of the soaked enchilada sauce zucchini (similar to lasagna making).

9. When needed, cover with the remaining cheese and olives on top—bake for 35 to 40 minutes.

10. Keep an eye on them.

11. When the cheese starts getting golden, cover with foil.

12. Serve and enjoy!

Nutrition:

- Calories: 312 Cal
- Carbohydrates: 21.3g
- Protein: 27g
- Fat: 10.2g

14. Salmon Feta and Pesto Wrap

Preparation Time: 15 Minutes

Cooking Time: 10 Minutes

Servings: 4

Ingredients:

- 8 Ounces (250g) smoked salmon fillet, thinly sliced
- 1 Cup (150g) feta cheese
- 8 (15g) Romaine lettuce leaves
- 4 (6-inch) Pita bread
- 1/4 Cup (60g) basil pesto sauce

Directions:

1. Place one pita bread on a plate. Top with lettuce, salmon, feta cheese, and pesto sauce. Fold or roll to enclose filling. Repeat the procedure for the remaining ingredients.
2. Serve and enjoy.

Nutrition:

- Calories: 379
- Fat: 17.7g
- Carbohydrates: 36.6g
- Protein: 18.4g
- Sodium: 554mg

15. Pan-Fried Trout

Preparation Time: 15 Minutes

Cooking Time: 10 Minutes

Servings: 4

Ingredients:

- 1 ¼ Pounds trout fillets
- 1/3 Cup white, or yellow, cornmeal
- ¼ Teaspoon anise seeds
- ¼ Teaspoon black pepper
- ½ Cup minced cilantro, or parsley
- Vegetable cooking spray
- Lemon wedges

Directions:

1. Coat the fish with combined cornmeal, spices, and cilantro, pressing them gently into the fish. Spray a large skillet with cooking spray; heat over medium heat until hot.

2. Add fish and cook until it is tender and flakes with a fork, about 5 minutes on each side. Serve with lemon wedges.

Nutrition:

- Calories: 207
- Total Carbohydrates: 19g
- Cholesterol: 27mg
- Total Fat: 16g
- Fiber: 4g
- Protein: 18g

16. Glazed Bananas in Phyllo Nut Cups

Preparation Time: 30 Minutes

Cooking Time: 45 Minutes

Servings: 6 Servings

Ingredients:

- 3/4 Cups shelled pistachios
- ½ Cup sugar
- 1 Teaspoon. ground cinnamon
- 4 Sheets phyllo dough (14 inches x 9 inches)
- 1/4 Cup butter, melted

Sauce:

- 3/4 Cup butter, cubed
- 3/4 Cup packed brown sugar
- 3 Medium-firm bananas, sliced
- 1/4 Teaspoon. ground cinnamon
- 3 to 4 Cups vanilla ice cream

Directions:

1. Finely chop sugar and pistachios in a food processor; move to a bowl, then mix in cinnamon. Slice each phyllo sheet into six four-inch squares, get rid of the trimmings. Pile the squares, then use plastic wrap to cover.

2. Slather melted butter on each square one at a time, then scatter a heaping tablespoonful of pistachio mixture. Pile three squares, flip each at an angle to misalign the corners. Force each stack on the sides and bottom of an oiled eight ounces custard cup. Bake for 15-20 minutes in a 350 degrees F oven until golden; cool for 5 minutes. Move to a wire rack to cool completely.

3. Melt and boil brown sugar and butter in a saucepan to make the sauce; lower heat. Mix in cinnamon and bananas gently; heat completely. Put ice cream in the phyllo cups until full, then put banana sauce on top. Serve right away.

Nutrition:

- Calories: 735
- Total Carbohydrate: 82g
- Cholesterol: 111mg
- Total Fat: 45g
- Fiber: 3g
- Protein: 7g
- Sodium: 468mg

17. Salmon Cream Cheese and Onion on Bagel

Preparation Time: 15 Minutes

Cooking Time: 10 Minutes

Servings: 4

Ingredients:

- 8 Ounces (250g) smoked salmon fillet, thinly sliced
- ½ Cup (125g) cream cheese
- 1 Medium (110g) onion, thinly sliced
- 4 Bagels (about 80g each), split
- 2 Tablespoons (7g) fresh parsley, chopped
- Freshly ground black pepper, to taste

Directions:

4. Spread the cream cheese on each bottom's half of bagels. Top with salmon and onion, season with pepper, sprinkle with parsley and then cover with bagel tops.

5. Serve and enjoy.

Nutrition:

- Calories: 309
- Fat: 14.1g
- Carbohydrates: 32.0g
- Protein: 14.7g
- Sodium: 571mg

18. Salmon Apple Salad Sandwich

Preparation Time: 15 Minutes

Cooking Time: 10 Minutes

Servings: 4

Ingredients:

- 4 Ounces (125g) canned pink salmon, drained and flaked
- 1 Medium (180g) red apple, cored and diced
- 1 Celery stalk (about 60g), chopped
- 1 Shallot (about 40g), finely chopped
- 1/3 Cup (85g) light mayonnaise
- 8 Whole grain bread slices (about 30g each), toasted
- 8 (15g) Romaine lettuce leaves
- Salt and freshly ground black pepper

Directions:

1. Combine the salmon, apple, celery, shallot, and mayonnaise in a mixing bowl—season with salt and pepper.
2. Place one bread slice on a plate, top with lettuce and salmon salad, and then cover it with another slice of bread—repeat the procedure for the remaining ingredients.
3. Serve and enjoy.

Nutrition:

- Calories: 315
- Fat: 11.3g
- Carbohydrates: 40.4g
- Protein: 15.1g
- Sodium: 469mg

19. Greek Baklava

Preparation Time: 20 Minutes

Cooking Time: 20 Minutes

Servings: 18

Ingredients:

- 1 (16 oz.) Package phyllo dough
- 1 lb. Chopped nuts
- 1 Cup butter
- 1 Teaspoon ground cinnamon
- 1 Cup water
- 1 Cup white sugar
- 1 Teaspoon vanilla extract
- ½ Cup honey

Directions:

1. Preheat the oven to 175°C or 350°Fahrenheit. Spread butter on the sides and bottom of a 9- by 13-inch pan.

2. Chop the nuts, then mix with cinnamon; set it aside. Unfurl the phyllo dough, then halve the whole stack to fit the pan. Use a damp cloth to cover the phyllo to prevent drying as you proceed. Put two phyllo sheets in the pan, then butter well. Repeat to make eight layered phyllo sheets. Scatter 2-3 tablespoons of the

nut mixture over the sheets, then place two more phyllo sheets on top, butter, sprinkle with nuts—layer as you go. The final layer should be six to eight phyllo sheets deep.

3. Make square or diamond shapes with a sharp knife up to the bottom of the pan. You can slice into four long rows for diagonal shapes. Bake until crisp and golden for 50 minutes.

4. Meanwhile, boil water and sugar until the sugar melts to make the sauce; mix in honey and vanilla. Let it simmer for 20 minutes.

5. Take the baklava out of the oven, then drizzle with sauce right away; cool. Serve the baklava in cupcake papers. You can also freeze them without cover. The baklava will turn soggy when wrapped.

Nutrition:

- Calories: 393
- Total Carbohydrate: 37.5g
- Cholesterol: 27mg
- Total Fat: 25.9g
- Protein: 6.1g
- Sodium: 196mg

20. Easy Salmon Burger

Preparation Time: 15 minutes

Cooking Time: 15 minutes

Servings: 6

Ingredients:

- 16 Ounces (450g) pink salmon, minced
- 1 Cup (250g) prepared mashed potatoes
- 1 Medium (110g) onion, chopped
- 1 Stalk celery (about 60g), finely chopped
- 1 Large egg (about 60g), lightly beaten
- 2 Tablespoons (7g) fresh cilantro, chopped
- 1 Cup (100g) breadcrumbs
- Vegetable oil, for deep frying
- Salt and freshly ground black pepper

Directions:

1. Combine the salmon, mashed potatoes, onion, celery, egg, and cilantro in a mixing bowl. Season to taste and mix thoroughly. Spoon about 2 Tablespoons of the mixture, roll in breadcrumbs, and then form into small patties.

2. Heat oil in a non-stick frying pan. Cook your salmon patties for 5 minutes on each side or until golden brown and crispy.

3. Serve in burger buns and with coleslaw on the side if desired.

4. Enjoy.

Nutrition:

- Calories: 230
- Fat: 7.9g
- Carbs: 20.9g
- Protein: 18.9g
- Sodium: 298mg

21. White Bean Dip

Preparation Time: 10 Minutes

Cooking Time: 0 Minutes

Servings: 4

Ingredients:

- 15 Ounces canned white beans, drained and rinsed
- 6 Ounces canned artichoke hearts, drained and quartered
- 4 Garlic cloves, minced
- 1 Tablespoon basil, chopped
- 2 Tablespoons olive oil
- Juice of ½ lemon
- Zest of ½ lemon, grated
- Salt and black pepper to the taste

Directions:

1. In your food processor, combine the beans with the artichokes and the rest of the ingredients except the oil and pulse well.
2. Add the oil gradually, pulse the mix again, divide into cups and serve as a party dip.

Nutrition:

- Calories: 274
- Fat: 11.7g
- Fiber: 6.5g
- Carbs: 18.5g
- Protein: 16.5g

22. Grilled Salmon Burger

Preparation Time: 15 Minutes

Cooking Time: 10 Minutes

Servings: 4

Ingredients:

- 16 Ounces (450g) pink salmon fillet, minced
- 1 Cup (250g) prepared mashed potatoes
- 1 Shallot (about 40g), chopped
- 1 Large egg (about 60g), lightly beaten
- 2 Tablespoons (7g) fresh coriander, chopped
- 4 Hamburger buns (about 60g each), split
- 1 Large tomato (about 150g), sliced
- 8 (15g) Romaine lettuce leaves
- 1/4 Cup (60g) mayonnaise
- Salt and freshly ground black pepper
- Cooking oil spray

Directions:

1. Combine the salmon, mashed potatoes, shallot, egg, and coriander in a mixing bowl—season with salt and pepper.
2. Spoon about two tablespoons of mixture and form into patties.

3. Preheat your grill or griddle on high—grease with cooking oil spray.
4. Grill the salmon patties for 4-5 minutes on each side or until cooked through. Transfer to a clean plate and cover to keep warm.
5. Spread some mayonnaise on the bottom half of the buns. Top with lettuce, salmon patty, and tomato. Cover with bun tops.
6. Serve and enjoy.

Nutrition:

- Calories: 395
- Fat: 18.0g
- Carbohydrates: 38.8g
- Protein: 21.8g
- Sodium: 383mg

23. Grilled Avocado Capers Crostini

Preparation Time: 10 Minutes

Cooking Time: 20 Minutes

Servings: 2

Ingredients:

- 1 Avocado thinly sliced
- 9 Ounces ripened cherry tomatoes
- 1.50 Ounces fresh bocconcini in water
- 2 Tsp. Balsamic glaze
- 8 Pieces Italian baguette
- ½ Cup basil leaves

Directions:

1. Preheat your oven to 375 degrees Fahrenheit
2. Arrange your baking sheet properly before spraying them on top with olive oil.
3. Cut and bake your baguette until golden brown. Rub your crostini with the cut side of garlic while they are still warm, and you can season them with pepper and salt.
4. Divide the basil leaves on each piece of bread and top them up with tomato halves, avocado slices, and bocconcini. Season it with pepper and salt.

5. Broil it for 4 minutes, and when the cheese starts to melt through, remove and drizzle balsamic glaze before serving.

Nutrition:

- Calories: 278
- Fat: 10g
- Carbohydrates: 37g
- Proteins: 10g
- Sodium: 342mg
- Potassium: 277mg

24. Cheesy Garlic Sweet Potatoes

Preparation Time: 10 Minutes

Cooking Time: 25 Minutes

Servings: 4

Ingredients:

- Sea salt
- ¼ Cup garlic butter melt
- ¾ Cup shredded mozzarella cheese
- ½ Cup of parmesan cheese freshly grated
- 4 Medium sized sweet potatoes
- 2 Tsp. freshly chopped parsley

Directions:

1. Heat the oven to 400 degrees Fahrenheit and brush the potatoes with garlic butter, and season each with pepper and salt. Arrange the cut side down on a greased baking sheet until the flesh is tender or they turn golden brown.

2. Remove them from the oven, flip the cut side up and top up with parsley and parmesan cheese.

3. Change the settings of your instant fryer oven to broil and on medium heat, add the cheese and melt it. Sprinkle salt and pepper to taste. Serve them warm.

Nutrition:

- Calories: 356
- Fat: 9g
- Carbohydrates: 13g
- Proteins: 5g
- Potassium: 232mg
- Sodium: 252mg

25. Crispy Garlic Baked Potato Wedges

Preparation Time: 5 Minutes

Cooking Time: 10 Minutes

Servings: 3

Ingredients:

- 3 Tsp. salt
- 1 Tsp. minced garlic
- 6 Large russet
- ¼ Cup olive oil
- 1 Tsp. Paprika
- 2/3 Finely grated parmesan cheese
- 2 Tsp. Freshly chopped parsley

Directions:

1. Preheat the oven to 350 degrees Fahrenheit and line the baking sheet with parchment paper.
2. Cut the potatoes into half-length and cut each half in half lengthways again. Make eight wedges.
3. In a small jug, combine garlic, oil, paprika, and salt and place your wedges in the baking sheets. Pour the oil mixture over the potatoes and toss them to ensure that they are evenly coated.

4. Arrange the potato wedges in a single layer on the baking tray and sprinkle salt and parmesan cheese if needed. Bake for 35 minutes and turn the wedges once half side is cooked.
5. Flip the other side until they are both golden brown.
6. Sprinkle parsley and the remaining parmesan before serving.

Nutrition:

- Calories: 324
- Fat: 6g
- Carbs: 8g
- Proteins: 2g
- Sodium: 51mg
- Potassium: 120mg

26. Cheesy Mashed Sweet Potato Cakes

Preparation Time: 10 Minutes

Cooking Time: 30 Minutes

Servings: 4

Ingredients:

- ¾ Cup bread crumbs
- 4 Cups mashed potatoes
- ½ Cup onions
- 2 Cup of grated mozzarella cheese
- ¼ Cup fresh grated parmesan cheese
- 2 Large garlic cloves finely chopped
- 1 Egg
- 2 Tsp. Finely chopped parsley
- Salt and pepper to taste

Directions:

1. Line your baking sheet with foil. Wash, peel and cut the sweet potatoes into six pieces. Arrange them inside the baking sheet and drizzle a small amount of oil on top before seasoning with salt and pepper.

2. Cover with a baking sheet and bake it for 45 minutes; once cooked, transfer them into a mixing bowl and mash them well with a potato masher.

3. Put the sweet potatoes in a bowl, add green onions, parmesan, mozzarella, garlic, egg, parsley, and bread crumbs. Mash and combine the mixture together using the masher.

4. Put the remaining ¼ cup of the breadcrumbs in place. Scoop a teaspoon of the mixture into your palm and form round patties around ½ an inch thick. Dredge your patties in the breadcrumbs to cover both sides and set them aside.

5. Heat a tablespoon of oil in a medium nonstick pan. When the oil is hot, begin to cook the patties in batches 4 or 5 per session and cook each side for 6 minutes until they turn golden brown. Use a spoon or spatula to flip them. Add oil to prevent burning.

Nutrition:
- Calories:126
- Fat:6g
- Carbs: 15g
- Proteins 3g
- Sodium: 400mg

27. Sticky Chicken Thai Wings

Preparation Time: 10 Minutes

Cooking Time: 30 Minutes

Servings: 6

Ingredients:

- 3 Pounds chicken wings removed
- 1 Tsp. sea salt to taste

For the glaze:

- ¾ Cup Thai sweet chili sauce
- ¼ Cup soy sauce
- 4 Tsp. brown sugar
- 4 Tsp. rice wine vinegar
- 3 Tsp. fish sauce
- 2 Tsp. lime juice
- 1 Tsp. lemongrass minced
- 2 Tsp. sesame oil
- 1 Tsp. garlic minced

Directions:

1. Preheat the oven to 350 degrees Fahrenheit. Lightly spray your baking tray with the cooking spray and set it aside. To prepare the glaze, combine the ingredients

in a small bowl and whisk them until they are well combined. Pour half of the mixture into a pan and reserve the rest.

2. Trim any excess skin off the wing edges and season it with pepper and salt. Add the wings to a baking tray and pour the sauce over the wings tossing them for the sauce to coat evenly. Arrange them in a single layer and bake them for 15 minutes.

3. While the wings are in the oven, bring your glaze to simmer in medium heat until there are visible bubbles.

4. Once the wings are cooked on one side, rotate each piece and bake for an extra 10 minutes. Baste them and return them into the oven to allow for more cooking until they are golden brown. Garnish with onion slices, cilantro, chili flakes, and sprinkle the remaining salt. Serve with some glaze as you desire.

Nutrition:
- Calories: 256
- Fat: 16g
- Carbohydrates 19g
- Proteins: 20g
- Potassium: 213mg
- Sodium: 561mg

28. Caprese Stuffed Garlic Butter Portobellos

Preparation Time: 5 Minutes

Cooking Time: 10 Minutes

Servings: 6

Ingredients:

For the garlic butter:

- 2 Tsp. of butter
- 2 Cloves garlic
- 1 Tsp. parsley finely chopped

For the mushrooms:

- 6 Large portobello mushrooms, washed and dried well with a paper towel
- 6 Mozzarella cheese balls thinly sliced
- 1 Cup grape tomatoes thinly sliced
- Fresh basil for garnishing

For the balsamic glaze:

- 2 Tsp. brown sugar
- ¼ Cup balsamic vinegar

Directions:

1. Preheat the oven to broil, setting on high heat. Arrange the oven shelf and place it in the right direction.

2. Combine the garlic butter ingredients in a small pan and melt until the garlic begins to be fragrant. Brush the bottoms of the mushroom and place them on the buttered section of the baking tray.

3. Flip and brush the remaining garlic over each cap. Fill each mushroom with tomatoes and mozzarella slices and grill until the cheese has melted. Drizzle the balsamic glaze and sprinkle some salt to taste.

4. If you are making the balsamic glaze from scratch, combine the sugar and vinegar in a small pan and reduce the heat to low. Allow it to simmer for 6 minutes or until the mixture has thickened well.

Nutrition:

- Calories: 101
- Fat: 5g
- Carbohydrates: 12g
- Proteins: 2g
- Sodium: 58mg
- Potassium: 377mg

29. Veggie Fritters

Preparation Time: 10 Minutes

Cooking Time: 10 Minutes

Servings: 4

Ingredients:

- 2 Garlic cloves, minced
- 2 Yellow onions, chopped
- 4 Scallions, chopped
- 2 Carrots, grated
- 2 Teaspoons cumin, ground
- ½ Teaspoon turmeric powder
- Salt and black pepper to the taste
- ¼ Teaspoon coriander, ground
- 2 Tablespoons parsley, chopped
- ¼ Teaspoon lemon juice
- ½ Cup almond flour
- 2 Beets, peeled and grated
- 2 Eggs, whisked
- ¼ Cup tapioca flour
- 3 Tablespoons olive oil

Directions:

1. In a bowl, combine the garlic with the onions, scallions, and the rest of the ingredients except the oil; stir well and shape medium fritters out of this mix.

2. Heat up a pan with the oil over medium-high heat, add the fritters, cook for 5 minutes on each side, arrange on a platter and serve.

Nutrition:

- Calories: 209
- Fat: 11.2g
- Fiber: 3g
- Carbs: 4.4g
- Protein: 4.8g

30. Eggplant Dip

Preparation Time: 10 Minutes

Cooking Time: 40 Minutes

Servings: 4

Ingredients:

- 1 Eggplant, poked with a fork
- 2 Tablespoons tahini paste
- 2 Tablespoons lemon juice
- 2 Garlic cloves, minced
- 1 Tablespoon olive oil
- Salt and black pepper to the taste
- 1 Tablespoon parsley, chopped

Directions:

1. Put the eggplant in a roasting pan, bake at 400°F for 40 minutes, cool down, peel, and transfer to your food processor.

2. Add the rest of the ingredients except the parsley, pulse well, divide into small bowls and serve as an appetizer with the parsley sprinkled on top.

Nutrition:

- Calories: 121
- Fat: 4.3g
- Fiber: 1g
- Carbs: 1.4g
- Protein:4.3g

32. Grandma's Rice

Preparation Time: 15 Minutes

Cooking Time: 2 Hours

Servings: 4

Ingredients:

- 40g Butter
- ½ Cup brown sugar
- ½ Cup arborio rice
- 3 Cups milk
- ½ Tbsp. ground cinnamon
- 1/8 Tbsp. ground nutmeg
- 1 Tbsp. vanilla paste
- ½ Cup raisins
- 300ml. Cream

Directions:

3. Preheat oven to 300°F.
4. Grease a 1-liter ability oven-safe plate.
5. Heat butter in a saucepan and add sugar and rice.
6. Stir for 1 minute to thoroughly coat the rice.
7. Remove from heat and wish in milk, spices, and vanilla.
8. Stir through raisins, then pour into the prepared dish.
9. Bake for 30 minutes, then remove from the oven and stir well.

10. Drizzle over the cream and return to the oven for an additional hour.

11. Check that the rice is cooked through.

12. Return to the oven for 15-30 minutes if required.

13. Serve with extra cream and nutmeg.

Nutrition:

- Fat: 20g
- Protein: 23g
- Cholesterol: 25mg
- Carbohydrates: 30g
- Sodium: 1000mg

33. Baked Beef Zucchini

Preparation Time: 10 Minutes

Cooking Time: 40 Minutes

Servings: 4

Ingredients:

- 2 Large zucchinis
- 1 Cup minced beef
- 1 Cup mushrooms, chopped
- 1 Tomato, chopped
- ½ Cup spinach, chopped
- 1 Tbsp. chives, minced
- 2 Tbsp. olive oil
- Salt and pepper to taste
- 1 Tbsp. almond butter
- 1 Tsp. garlic powder
- 1 Cup cheddar cheese, grated
- 1/3 Tsp. ginger powder

Directions:

1. Preheat the oven to 400 degrees F.
2. Add aluminum foil on a baking sheet.
3. Cut the zucchini in half. Scoop out the seeds and make pockets to stuff them later.

4. In a pan, add the olive oil.

5. Toss the beef until brown.

6. Add the mushrooms, tomato, chives, salt, pepper, garlic, ginger, and spinach.

7. Cook for 2 minutes. Take off the heat.

8. Stuff the zucchinis using the mix.

9. Add them onto the baking sheet. Sprinkle the cheese on top.

10. Add the butter on top—bake for 30 minutes. Serve warm.

Nutrition:
- Fat: 12.8g
- Cholesterol: 79.7mg
- Sodium: 615.4mg
- Potassium: 925.8mg
- Carbohydrate: 26.8g

34. Nutmeg Nougat

Preparation Time: 30 Minutes

Cooking Time: 60 Minutes

Servings: 12

Ingredients:

- 1 Cup heavy cream
- 1 Cup cashew butter
- 1 Cup coconut, shredded
- ½ Teaspoon nutmeg
- 1 Teaspoon vanilla extract, pure
- Stevia to taste

Directions:

1. Melt your cashew butter using a double boiler, and then stir in your vanilla extract, dairy cream, nutmeg, and stevia. Make sure it's mixed well.

2. Remove from heat, allowing it to cool down before refrigerating it for half an hour.

3. Shape into balls, and coat with shredded coconut. Chill for at least two hours before serving.

Nutrition:

- Calories: 341
- Fat: 34g
- Carbohydrates: 5g

35. Baked Tuna With Asparagus

Preparation Time: 10 Minutes

Cooking Time: 10 Minutes

Servings: 2

Ingredients:

- 2 Tuna steak
- 1 Cup asparagus, trimmed
- 1 Tsp. almond butter
- 1 Tsp. rosemary
- ½ Tsp. oregano
- ½ Tsp. garlic powder
- 1 Tsp. lemon juice
- ½ Tsp. ginger powder
- 1 Tbsp. olive oil
- 1 Tsp. red chili powder
- Salt and pepper to taste

Directions:

1. Marinate the tuna using oregano, lemon juice, salt, pepper, red chili powder, garlic, ginger, and let it sit for 10 minutes.
2. In a pan, add the olive oil.
3. Fry the tuna steaks for 2 minutes per side.
4. In another pan, melt the almond butter.

5. Toss the asparagus with salt, pepper, and rosemary for 3 minutes.

6. Serve.

Nutrition:

- Fat: 4.7g
- Cholesterol: 0.0mg
- Sodium: 98.5mg
- Potassium: 171.6mg
- Carbohydrate: 3.2g

36. Chocolate Orange Bites

Preparation Time: 20 Minutes

Cooking Time: 120 Minutes

Servings: 6

Ingredients:

- 10 Ounces coconut oil
- 4 Tablespoons cocoa powder
- ¼ Teaspoon orange extract
- Stevia to taste

Directions:

1. Melt half of your coconut oil using a double boiler, and then add in your stevia and orange extract.

2. Get out candy molds, pouring the mixture into them. Fill each mold halfway, and then place them in the fridge until they set.

3. Melt the other half of your coconut oil, stirring in your cocoa powder and stevia, making sure that the mixture is smooth with no lumps.

4. Pour into your molds, filling them up all the way, and then allow it to set in the fridge before serving.

Nutrition:

- Calories: 188g
- Protein: 1g
- Fat: 21g
- Carbohydrates: 5g

37. Goat Cheese and Chives Spread

Preparation Time: 10 Minutes

Cooking Time: 0 Minute

Servings: 4

Ingredients:

- 2 Ounces goat cheese, crumbled
- ¾ Cup sour cream
- 2 Tablespoons chives, chopped
- 1 Tablespoon lemon juice
- Salt and black pepper to the taste
- 2 Tablespoons extra virgin olive oil

Directions:

1. In a bowl, mix the goat cheese with the cream and the rest of the ingredients and whisk very well.
2. Keep in the fridge for 10 minutes and serve as a party spread.

Nutrition:

- Calories: 220
- Fat: 11.5g
- Fiber: 4.8g
- Carbs: 8.9g
- Protein: 5.6g

38. Jalapeno Lentil Burgers

Preparation Time: 15 Minutes
Cooking Time: 10 Minutes
Servings: 5

Ingredients:
- Half cup dried red lentils, rinsed
- 1 to 12 Ounces can Chickpeas, rinsed
- 1 Teaspoon Ground cumin
- 1 Teaspoon Chili powder
- 1 Teaspoon Sea salt
- Half cup Packed cilantro
- ½ Teaspoon Garlic cloves minced
- 1 Teaspoon Jalapeno finely chopped
- Red onion; half, small; minced
- 1 cup chopped Red bell pepper
- ¾ cup Carrot; shredded
- 1/4 Cup Oat bran/oat flour (gluten-free)
- Lettuce/hamburger buns

For the Pico:
- Ripe mango (1) diced
- Ripe avocado (1) diced
- Red onion; half, small; finely diced
- Chopped cilantro; half cup
- Fresh lime juice; half teaspoon
- Sea salt

Directions:

1. For the pico, put all ingredients in a large bowl and mix.
2. Stir in the salt to taste.
3. Put a medium saucepan on medium heat, add lentils plus 1 ½ cups of water, then bring water to a boil, cover it afterward, lower the heat to low, and then simmer lentils until the water is absorbed.
4. Drain, and set aside some extra water.
5. In a food processor, put the cooked lentils, chickpeas, garlic, sea salt, cilantro, chili powder, and cumin, and blend until the beans and lentils are smooth.
6. Add tomato, red pepper, jalapeno, and carrot to process.
7. Divide into six equal parts and use your hands to create dense patties.
8. Heat skillet over a medium-high flame; apply ½ tablespoon of olive oil
9. Place a few burgers in at a time and cook on either side for a couple of minutes, just until crisp and golden brown.
10. Repeat with remaining patties and add olive oil whenever desired.
11. Place the patties in a bun or lettuce and finish with mango avocado pico.

Nutrition:

- Carbohydrates: 34.9g
- Calories: 225 Cal
- Sugar: 7.7g
- Fats: 6.1g

39. Cocoa Brownies

Preparation Time: 10 Minutes

Cooking Time: 30 Minutes

Servings: 12

Ingredients:

- 1 Egg
- 2 Tablespoons butter, grass-fed
- 2 Teaspoons vanilla extract, pure
- ¼ Teaspoon baking powder
- ¼ Cup cocoa powder
- 1/3 Cup heavy cream
- ¾ Cup almond butter
- Pinch sea salt

Directions:

1. Break your egg into a bowl, whisking until smooth.
2. Add in all of your wet ingredients, mixing well.
3. Mix all dry ingredients into a bowl.
4. Sift your dry ingredients into your wet ingredients, mixing to form a batter.
5. Use a baking pan, greasing it before pouring in your mixture.
6. Heat your oven to 350 and bake for twenty-five minutes.
7. Allow it to cool before slicing and serve at room temperature or warm.

Nutrition:

- Calories: 184
- Protein: 1g
- Fat: 20g
- Carbohydrates: 1g

40. Avocado Dip

Preparation Time: 5 Minutes

Cooking Time: 0 Minutes

Servings: 8

Ingredients:

- ½ Cup heavy cream
- 1 Green chili pepper, chopped
- Salt and pepper to the taste
- 4 Avocados, pitted, peeled, and chopped
- 1 Cup cilantro, chopped
- ¼ Cup lime juice

Directions:

1. In a blender, combine the cream with the avocados and the rest of the ingredients and pulse well.
2. Divide the mix into bowls and serve cold as a party dip.

Nutrition:

- Calories: 200
- Fat: 14.5g
- Fiber: 3.8g
- Carbs: 8.1g
- Protein: 7.6g

41. Mediterranean Chicken Salad

Preparation Time: 15 Minutes

Cooking Time: 30 Minutes

Servings: 4

Ingredients:

For the Chicken:

- 1 3/4 lb. Boneless, skinless chicken breast
- 1/4 Teaspoon each of pepper and salt (or as desired)
- 1 ½ Tablespoon of butter, melted

For the Mediterranean Salad:

- 1 Cup of sliced cucumber
- 6 Cups of romaine lettuce, torn or roughly chopped
- 10 Pitted Kalamata olives
- 1 Pint of cherry tomatoes
- 1/3 Cup of reduced-fat feta cheese
- 1/4 Teaspoon each of pepper and salt (or lesser)
- 1 Small lemon juice (It should be about 2 tablespoons)

Directions:

1. Preheat your oven or grill to about 350°F.

2. Season the chicken with salt, butter, and black pepper

3. Roast or grill chicken until it reaches an internal temperature of 165°F in about 25 minutes.

4. Once your chicken breasts are cooked, remove and keep them aside to rest for about 5 minutes before you slice them.

5. Combine all the salad ingredients you have and toss everything together very well.

6. Serve the chicken with a Mediterranean salad.

Nutrition:

- Calories: 340 Cal
- Protein: 45g
- Carbohydrates: 9g
- Fat: 14g

42. Avocado Taco Boats

Preparation Time: 5 Minutes

Cooking Time: 20 Minutes

Servings: 4

Ingredients:

- 4 Grape tomatoes
- 2 Large avocados
- 1 lb. Ground beef
- 4 Tablespoon taco seasoning
- 3/4 Cups shredded sharp cheddar cheese
- 4 Slices pickled jalapeño
- 1/4 Cup salsa
- 3 Shredded romaine leaves
- 1/4 Cup sour cream
- 2/3 Cups water

Directions:

1. Take a skillet of large size, grease it with oil, and heat it over medium-high heat. Cook the ground beef in it for 10-15 minutes or until it gives a brownish look.

2. Once the beef gets brown, drain the grease from the skillet and add the water and the taco seasoning.

3. Reduce the heat once the taco seasoning gets mixed well and simmer for 8-10 minutes.
4. Take both avocados and prepare their halves using a sharp knife.
5. Take each avocado shell and fill it with ¼ of the shredded romaine leaves.
6. Fill each shell with ¼ of the cooked ground beef.
7. Make the topping with sour cream, cheese, jalapeno, salsa, and tomatoes before you serve the delicious avocado taco boats.

Nutrition:

- Calories: 430
- Fat: 35g
- Carbohydrates: 5g
- Protein: 32g

43. Lamb Stuffed Avocado

Preparation Time: 10 Minutes

Cooking Time: 40 Minutes

Servings: 4

Ingredients:

- 2 Avocados
- 1 ½ Cup minced lamb
- ½ Cup cheddar cheese, grated
- ½ Cup parmesan cheese, grated
- 2 Tbsp. almond, chopped
- 1 Tbsp. coriander, chopped
- 2 Tbsp. olive oil
- 1 Tomato, chopped
- 1 Jalapeno, chopped
- Salt and pepper to taste
- 1 Tsp. garlic, chopped
- 1 Inch ginger, chopped

Directions:

1. Cut the avocados in half. Remove the pit and scoop out some flesh to stuff it later.
2. In a skillet, add half of the oil.
3. Toss the ginger, garlic for 1 minute.

4. Add the lamb and toss for 3 minutes.
5. Add the tomato, coriander, parmesan, jalapeno, salt, pepper, and cook for 2 minutes.
6. Take off the heat. Stuff the avocados.
7. Sprinkle the almonds, cheddar cheese, and add olive oil on top.
8. Add to a baking sheet and bake for 30 minutes. Serve.

Nutrition:

- Fat: 19.5g
- Cholesterol: 167.5mg
- Sodium: 410.7mg
- Potassium: 617.1mg
- Carbohydrate: 13.1g

44. Strawberry Cheesecake Minis

Preparation Time: 30 Minutes

Cooking Time: 120 Minutes

Servings: 12

Ingredients:

- 1 Cup coconut oil
- 1 Cup coconut butter
- ½ Cup strawberries, sliced
- ½ Teaspoon lime juice
- 2 Tablespoons cream cheese, full fat
- Stevia to taste

Directions:

1. Blend the strawberries.
2. Soften your cream cheese, and then add in your coconut butter.
3. Combine all ingredients together, and then pour your mixture into silicone molds.
4. Freeze for at least two hours before serving.

Nutrition:

- Calories: 372
- Protein: 1g
- Fat: 41g
- Carbohydrates: 2g

45. Coconut Fudge

Preparation Time: 20 Minutes

Cooking Time: 60 Minutes

Servings: 12

Ingredients:

- 2 Cups coconut oil
- ½ Cup dark cocoa powder
- ½ Cup coconut cream
- ¼ Cup almonds, chopped
- ¼ Cup coconut, shredded
- 1 Teaspoon almond extract
- Pinch of salt
- Stevia to taste

Directions:

1. Pour your coconut oil and coconut cream in a bowl, whisking with an electric beater until smooth. Once the mixture becomes smooth and glossy, do not continue.
2. Begin to add in your cocoa powder while mixing slowly, making sure that there are not any lumps.
3. Add in the rest of your ingredients, and mix well.
4. Line a pan with parchment paper, and freeze until it sets.
5. Slice into squares before serving.

Nutrition:

- Calories: 172
- Fat: 20g
- Carbohydrates: 3g

46. Cinnamon Bites

Preparation Time: 20 Minutes

Cooking Time: 95 Minutes

Servings: 6

Ingredients:

- 1/8 Teaspoon nutmeg
- 1 Teaspoon vanilla extract
- ¼ Teaspoon cinnamon
- 4 Tablespoons coconut oil
- ½ Cup butter, grass-fed
- 8 Ounces cream cheese
- Stevia to taste

Directions:

1. Soften your coconut oil and butter, mixing in your cream cheese.
2. Add all of your remaining ingredients, and mix well.
3. Pour into molds, and freeze until set.

Nutrition:

- Calories: 178
- Protein: 1g
- Fat: 19g

47. Sweet Almond Bites

Preparation Time: 30 Minutes

Cooking Time: 90 Minutes

Servings: 12

Ingredients:

- 18 Ounces butter, grass-fed
- 2 Ounces heavy cream
- ½ Cup Stevia
- 2/3 Cup cocoa powder
- 1 Teaspoon vanilla extract, pure
- 4 Tablespoons almond butter

Directions:

1. Use a double boiler to melt your butter before adding in all of your remaining ingredients.
2. Place the mixture into molds, freezing for two hours before serving.

Nutrition:

- Calories: 350
- Protein: 2g
- Fat: 38g

48. Fluffy Bites

Preparation Time: 20 Minutes

Cooking Time: 60 Minutes

Servings: 12

Ingredients:

- 2 Teaspoons cinnamon
- 2/3 Cup sour cream
- 2 Cups heavy cream
- 1 Teaspoon scraped vanilla bean
- ¼ Teaspoon cardamom
- 4 Egg yolks
- Stevia to taste

Directions:

1. Start by whisking your egg yolks until creamy and smooth.
2. Use a double boiler, and add your eggs with the rest of your ingredients. Mix well.
3. Remove from heat, allowing it to cool until it reaches room temperature.
4. Refrigerate for an hour before whisking well.
5. Pour into molds, and freeze for at least an hour before serving.

Nutrition:

- Calories: 363
- Protein: 2g
- Fat: 40g
- Carbohydrates: 1g

49. Caramel Cones

Preparation Time: 25 Minutes

Cooking Time: 120 Minutes

Servings: 6

Ingredients:

- 2 Tablespoons heavy whipping cream
- 2 Tablespoons sour cream
- 1 Tablespoon caramel sugar
- 1 Teaspoon sea salt, fine
- 1/3 Cup butter, grass-fed
- 1/3 Cup coconut oil
- Stevia to taste

Directions:

1. Soften your coconut oil and butter, mixing together.
2. Mix all ingredients to form a batter, and then place them in molds.
3. Top with a little salt, and keep refrigerated until serving.

Nutrition:

- Calories: 100
- Fat: 12g
- Carbohydrates: 1g

50. Easy Vanilla Bombs

Preparation Time: 20 Minutes

Cooking Time: 45 Minutes

Servings: 14

Ingredients:

- 1 Cup macadamia nuts, unsalted
- ¼ Cup coconut oil
- ¼ Cup butter
- 2 Teaspoons vanilla extract, sugar-free
- 20 Drops liquid Stevia
- 2 Tablespoons erythritol, powdered

Directions:

1. Pulse your macadamia nuts in a blender, and then combine all of your ingredients together. Mix well.
2. Use mini muffin tins with a tablespoon and pour the mixture.
3. Refrigerate it for half an hour before serving.

Nutrition:

- Calories: 125
- Fat: 5g
- Carbohydrates: 5g

51. Sweet Chai Bites

Preparation Time: 20 Minutes

Cooking Time: 45 Minutes

Servings: 6

Ingredients:

- 1 Cup cream cheese
- 1 Cup coconut oil
- 2 Ounces butter, grass-fed
- 2 Teaspoons ginger
- 2 Teaspoons cardamom
- 1 Teaspoon nutmeg
- 1 Teaspoon cloves
- 1 Teaspoon vanilla extract, pure
- 1 Teaspoon Darjeeling black tea
- Stevia to taste

Directions:

1. Melt your coconut oil and butter before adding in your black tea. Allow it to sit for one to two minutes.
2. Add in your cream cheese, removing your mixture from heat.
3. Add in all of your spices, and stir to combine.
4. Pour into molds, and freeze before serving.

Nutrition:

- Calories: 178
- Protein: 1g
- Fat: 19g

52. Mozzarella Sticks

Preparation Time: 8 Minutes

Cooking Time: 2 Minutes

Servings: 2

Ingredients:

- 1 Large whole egg
- 3 Sticks mozzarella cheese in half (frozen overnight)
- 2 Tablespoon grated parmesan cheese
- ½ Cup almond flour
- 1/4 Cup coconut oil
- 2 ½ Teaspoons Italian seasoning blend
- 1 Tablespoon chopped parsley
- ½ Teaspoon salt

Directions:

1. Heat the coconut oil in a cast-iron skillet of medium size over low-medium heat.
2. Crack the egg in a small bowl in the meantime and beat it well.
3. Take another bowl of medium size and add parmesan cheese, almond flour, and seasonings to it. Whisk together the ingredients until a smooth mixture is prepared.

4. Take the overnight frozen mozzarella sticks and dip them in the beaten egg, then coat well with the dry mixture. Do the same with all the remaining cheese sticks.

5. Place all the coated sticks in the preheated skillet and cook them for 2 minutes or until they start giving a golden-brown look from all sides.

6. Remove from the skillet once cooked properly and place over a paper towel so that any extra oil gets absorbed.

7. Sprinkle parsley over the sticks if you desire and serve with keto marinara sauce.

Nutrition:

- Calories: 430
- Fat: 39g
- Carbohydrates: 10g
- Protein: 20g

53. Bulgur Lamb Meatballs

Preparation Time: 10 Minutes

Cooking Time: 15 Minute

Servings: 6

Ingredients:

- 1 and ½ Cups Greek yogurt
- ½ Teaspoon cumin, ground
- 1 cup cucumber, shredded
- ½ Teaspoon garlic, minced
- A pinch of salt and black pepper
- 1 Cup bulgur
- 2 Cups water
- 1 Pound lamb, ground
- ¼ Cup parsley, chopped
- ¼ Cup shallots, chopped
- ½ Teaspoon allspice, ground
- ½ Teaspoon cinnamon powder
- 1 Tablespoon olive oil

Directions:

1. In a bowl, combine the bulgur with the water, cover the bowl, leave aside for 10 minutes, drain and transfer to a bowl.
2. Add the meat, the yogurt, and the rest of the ingredients except the oil, stir well and shape medium meatballs out of this mix.
3. Heat up a pan with the oil over medium-high heat, add the meatballs, cook them for 7 minutes on each side, arrange them all on a platter and serve as an appetizer.

Nutrition:

- Calories: 300
- Fat: 9.6g
- Fiber: 4.6g
- Carbs: 22.6g
- Protein: 6.6g

54. Greek Tuna Salad Bites

Preparation Time: 5 Minutes

Cooking Time: 10 Minutes

Servings: 6

Ingredients:

- 2 Medium Cucumbers
- 2 6 oz. Cans White tuna
- Half of 1 lemon juice
- .5 Cup Red bell pepper
- .25 Cup Sweet/red onion
- .25 Cup Black olives
- 2 Tablespoon Garlic
- 2 Tablespoon Olive oil
- 2 Tablespoon Fresh parsley
- Dried oregano, salt, pepper as desired

Directions:

1. Drain and flake the tuna. Juice the lemon. Dice/chop the onions, olives, pepper, parsley, and garlic cup. Slice each of the cucumbers into thick rounds (skin off or on).
2. In a mixing container, combine the rest of the ingredients.
3. Place a heaping spoonful of salad onto the rounds and enjoy for your next party or just a snack.

Nutrition:

- Calories: 400
- Fats: 22g
- Carbs: 26g
- Fiber: Content: 8g
- Protein: 30g

55. Olives and Cheese Stuffed Tomatoes

Preparation Time: 10 Minutes

Cooking Time: 0 Minutes

Servings: 24

Ingredients:

- 24 Cherry tomatoes, top cut off, and insides scooped out
- 2 Tablespoons olive oil
- ¼ Teaspoon red pepper flakes
- ½ Cup feta cheese, crumbled
- 2 Tablespoons black olive paste
- ¼ Cup mint, torn

Directions:

1. In a bowl, mix the olives paste with the rest of the ingredients except the cherry tomatoes and whisk well.
2. Stuff the cherry tomatoes with this mix, arrange them all on a platter, and serve as an appetizer.

Nutrition:

- Calories: 136
- Fat: 8.6g
- Fiber: 4.8g
- Carbs: 5.6g
- Protein: 5.1g

56. Feta Artichoke Dip

Preparation Time: 10 Minutes

Cooking Time: 30 Minutes

Servings: 8

Ingredients:

- 8 Ounces artichoke hearts, drained and quartered
- ¾ Cups basil, chopped
- ¾ Cups green olives, pitted and chopped
- 1 Cup parmesan cheese, grated
- 5 Ounces feta cheese, crumbled

Directions:

1. In your food processor, mix the artichokes with the basil and the rest of the ingredients, pulse well, and transfer to a baking dish.
2. Introduce in the oven, bake at 375°F for 30 minutes and serve as a party dip.

Nutrition:

- Calories: 186
- Fat: 12.4g
- Fiber: 0.9g
- Carbs: 2.6g
- Protein: 1.5g

57. Cucumber Rolls

Preparation Time: 5 Minutes

Cooking Time: 0 Minutes

Servings: 6

Ingredients:

- 1 Big cucumber, sliced lengthwise
- 1 Tablespoon parsley, chopped
- 8 Ounces canned tuna, drained and mashed
- Salt and black pepper to the taste
- 1 Teaspoon lime juice

Directions:

1. Arrange cucumber slices on a working surface, divide the rest of the ingredients among them, and roll.
2. Arrange all the rolls on a platter and serve as an appetizer.

Nutrition:

- Calories: 200
- Fat: 6g
- Fiber: 3.4g
- Carbs: 7.6g
- Protein: 3.5g

58. Chili Mango and Watermelon Salsa

Preparation Time: 5 Minutes

Cooking Time: 0 Minutes

Servings: 12

Ingredients:

- 1 Red tomato, chopped
- Salt and black pepper to the taste
- 1 Cup watermelon, seedless, peeled and cubed
- 1 Red onion, chopped
- 2 Mangos, peeled and chopped
- 2 Chili peppers, chopped
- ¼ Cup cilantro, chopped
- 3 Tablespoons lime juice
- Pita chips for serving

Directions:

1. In a bowl, mix the tomato with the watermelon, the onion, and the rest of the ingredients except the pita chips and toss well.

2. Divide the mix into small cups and serve with pita chips on the side.

Nutrition:

- Calories: 62
- Fat: 4g
- Fiber: 1.3g
- Carbs: 3.9g
- Protein: 2.3g

59. Cucumber Bites

Preparation Time: 10 Minutes

Cooking Time: 0 Minutes

Servings: 12

Ingredients:

- 1 English cucumber, sliced into 32 rounds
- 10 Ounces hummus
- 16 Cherry tomatoes, halved
- 1 Tablespoon parsley, chopped
- 1 Ounce feta cheese, crumbled

Directions:

1. Spread the hummus on each cucumber round, divide the tomato halves on each, sprinkle the cheese and parsley on to, and serve as an appetizer.

Nutrition:

- Calories: 162
- Fat: 3.4g
- Fiber: 2g
- Carbs: 6.4g
- Protein: 2.4g

60. Wrapped Plums

Preparation Time: 5 Minutes

Cooking Time: 0 Minutes

Servings: 8

Ingredients:

- 2 Ounces prosciutto, cut into 16 pieces
- 4 Plums, quartered
- 1 Tablespoon chives, chopped
- A pinch of red pepper flakes, crushed

Directions:

1. Wrap each plum quarter in a prosciutto slice, arrange them all on a platter, sprinkle the chives and pepper flakes all over, and serve.

Nutrition:

- Calories: 30
- Fat: 1g
- Fiber: 0g
- Carbs: 4g
- Protein: 2g

61. Tomato Salsa

Preparation Time: 5 Minutes

Cooking Time: 0 Minutes

Servings: 6

Ingredients:

- 1 Garlic clove, minced
- 4 Tablespoons olive oil
- 5 Tomatoes, cubed
- 1 Tablespoon balsamic vinegar
- ¼ Cup basil, chopped
- 1 Tablespoon parsley, chopped
- 1 Tablespoon chives, chopped
- Salt and black pepper to the taste
- Pita chips for serving

Directions:

1. In a bowl, mix the tomatoes with the garlic and the rest of the ingredients except the pita chips, stir, divide into small cups and serve with the pita chips on the side.

Nutrition:

- Calories: 160
- Fat: 13.7g
- Fiber: 5.5g
- Carbs: 10.1g
- Protein: 2.2

62. Cucumber Sandwich Bites

Preparation Time: 5 Minutes

Cooking Time: 0 Minutes

Servings: 12

Ingredients:

- 1 Cucumber, sliced
- 8 Slices whole wheat bread
- 2 Tablespoons cream cheese, soft
- 1 Tablespoon chives, chopped
- ¼ Cup avocado, peeled, pitted, and mashed
- 1 Teaspoon mustard
- Salt and black pepper to the taste

Directions:

1. Spread the mashed avocado on each bread slice, also spread the rest of the ingredients except the cucumber slices.
2. Divide the cucumber slices into the bread slices, cut each slice in thirds, arrange on a platter and serve as an appetizer.

Nutrition:

- Calories: 187
- Fat: 12.4g
- Fiber: 2.1g
- Carbs: 4.5g
- Protein: 8.2g

63. Creamy Spinach and Shallots Dip

Preparation Time: 10 Minutes

Cooking Time: 0 Minutes

Servings: 4

Ingredients:

- 1 Pound spinach, roughly chopped
- 2 Shallots, chopped
- 2 Tablespoons mint, chopped
- ¾ Cups cream cheese, soft
- Salt and black pepper to the taste

Directions:

1. In a blender, combine the spinach with the shallots and the rest of the ingredients, and pulse well.
2. Divide into small bowls and serve as a party dip.

Nutrition:

- Calories: 204
- Fat: 11.5g
- Fiber: 3.1g
- Carbs: 4.2g
- Protein: 5.9g

64. Hummus With Ground Lamb

Preparation Time: 10 Minutes
Cooking Time: 15 Minute
Servings: 8

Ingredients:
- 10 Ounces hummus
- 12 Ounces lamb meat, ground
- ½ Cup pomegranate seeds
- ¼ Cup parsley, chopped
- 1 Tablespoon olive oil
- Pita chips for serving

Directions:
1. Heat up a pan with the oil over medium-high heat, add the meat, and brown for 15 minutes, stirring often.
2. Spread the hummus on a platter, spread the ground lamb all over, also spread the pomegranate seeds and the parsley, and serve with pita chips as a snack.

Nutrition:
- Calories: 133
- Fat: 9.7g
- Fiber: 1.7g
- Carbs: 6.4g
- Protein: 5

65. Coconut Shrimp

Preparation Time: 15 Minutes

Cooking Time: 15 Minutes

Servings: 6

Ingredients:

- Salt and pepper
- 1-pound Jumbo shrimp peeled and deveined
- ½ Cup all-purpose flour

For the batter:

- ½ Cup beer
- 1 Tsp. Baking powder
- ½ Cup all-purpose flour
- 1 Egg

For the coating:

- 1 Cup panko bread crumbs
- 1 Cup shredded coconut

Directions:

1. Line the baking tray with parchment paper.
2. In a shallow bowl, add ½ cup flour for dredging, and in another bowl, whisk the batter ingredients. The batter should

resemble a pancake consistency. If it is too thick, add a little mineral or beer whisking in between; in another bowl, mix together the shredded coconut and bread crumbs.

3. Dredge the shrimps in flour, shaking off any excess before dipping in the batter, and coat them with the bread crumb mixture. Lightly press the coconut into the shrimp.

4. Place them into the baking sheet and repeat the process until you have several.

5. In a Dutch oven skillet, heat vegetable oil until it is nice and hot, fry the frozen shrimp batches for 3 minutes per side. Drain them on a paper towel-lined plate.

6. Serve immediately with sweet chili sauce.

Nutrition:

- Calories: 409
- Fat: 11g
- Carbohydrates: 46g
- Proteins: 30g
- Sodium: 767mg
- Potassium: 345mg

CPSIA information can be obtained
at www.ICGtesting.com
Printed in the USA
BVHW090850140621
609525BV00002B/85

9 781914 599422